# FIGHTING CANCER NATURALLY:

*The Extraordinary Stories Of The Researcher Who Has Cured Himself And Helped His Friend Cure Cancer Miraculously!*

**DONG LA**

inside this book. You agree that by continuing to read this book, where appropriate and/or necessary, you shall consult a professional (including but not limited to your doctor, attorney, or financial advisor or such other advisor as needed) before using any of the suggested remedies, techniques, or information in this book.

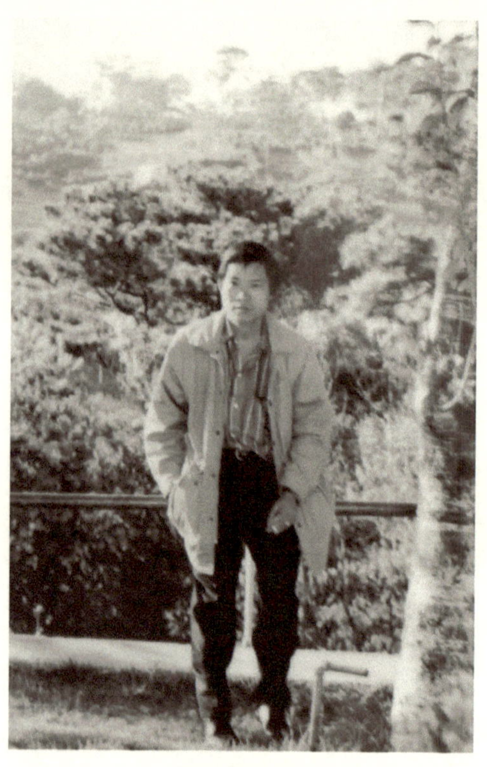

**-DONG LA-**

**(Writer and Pharmaceutical Chemical Researcher)**

# TABLE OF CONTENT


INTRODUCTION ..................................................................................6

PART I: 5 EXTRAORDINARY STORIES BUT TRUE IN THE FIGHT AGAINST CANCER ...................................................................9

Story Nº 1: The writer who used to be a pharmaceutical chemical researcher has cured himself and helped his friend cure cancer ........................................10

Story Nº 2: Seeing the friend with liver cancer ..................................16

The story Nº3: The doctor, a director of a hospital in the US that eats vegetarian food to cure cancer ........................................................26

Story Nº4: The man who fasted and ate vegetarian food won the battle against cancer .....................................................................................32

Story Nº5: The 93-year-old Chinese woman has beaten cancer for 44 years ......................................................................................................37

PART II: THE "MACROBIOTIC" DIET ...........................................39

**George Ohsawa** ..................................................................................40

PART III: THE SCIENTIFIC NATURE OF THE VEGETARIANISM TO CURE CANCER ...........................................44

The harmful effects of eating too much animal meat ........................45

The tumor died of its greediness! ......................................................51

The metabolism in the body ..............................................................56

The free radicals ................................................................................63

The protein synthesis in cell ..............................................................67

American eating habits and the status of their illnesses ....................69

**DISCUSSION** ......................................................................................71

Appendix ............................................................................................72

The story about a "Holy Lady" which has a strange ability to cure cancer .72

# INTRODUCTION

In this book, there are 5 stories of people who defeat cancer with a vegetarian diet including the author of this book. They are extraordinary stories, but they are completely true.

In fact, many people who were healed by this vegetarian diet, but modern medicine still did not believe it. Therefore, it has not been thoroughly researched yet, and it is still too far to be applied even if the hospitals failed to treat cancer for the patients.

Doctors usually thought that if patients ate protein from plant sources instead of animal protein in a vegetarian diet, their body would lack amino acids, especially essential amino acids. However, in fact, vegetarians are not only healthy but also cured of many diseases, including cancer. This is understandable because eating a plant food source may lack some essential amino acids, but if patients eat a variety of foods, they will get all they need.

Unfortunately, the numbers of people get sick and dying from cancer is still constantly increasing. The Doctors in the hospitals remain helpless when cancer patients are found to be late and cancer prevention and treatment with diet is still difficult and not good. Because of eating habits, it is difficult for people to follow a proper and enough vegetarian diet to cure cancer. Without understanding the scientific nature of vegetarianism to cure cancer, people will also apply it no well.

Therefore, when there is no other way, between death and a vegetarian diet, one is forced to choose vegetarianism; and for a vegetarian to cure cancer effectively, one must have knowledge. The people who have won the battle against cancer in this book are like that.

***

As a researcher in the field of pharmaceutical chemistry, I find that the deepest nature of a vegetarian diet against cancer is the need to eliminate the supply of nutrients to the tumor. I personally see the tumor that like a plant sprout, so it grows stronger than the cells of body. It needs nutrition many times more than the body's normal requirements. In the daily diet, if the cancer patient consumes more protein than the body's needs, this excess protein will be a source of nutrients for the growth of the tumor. But why do cancer patients eat plant protein instead of animal protein that can cure cancer?

The human body cannot directly use protein from food to perform functions. Once the protein is eaten in the stomach, the digestive process will take place. The large protein molecules will be hydrolyzed into amino acids. These amino acids are the material for cells in the human body to synthesize proteins. These proteins perform the functions of the body, including the building of musculoskeletal systems. Sadly for cancer patients, the cancer cells also use those amino acids to synthesize proteins to growing tumors. Conversely, if the cancer patients eat plant proteins instead of animal proteins, they will avoid the harmful effects of that excess because plant proteins are proteins that contain little amount of essential amino acids. The essential amino acids are acids that the human body cannot synthesize on its own. If the protein synthesis lacks only one essential amino acid, the whole string of protein molecules will be not formed. The cancer cells will not synthesize the protein to provide for the growth of the tumor; it will die, and finally, the patient is the winner!

Therefore, although the patient does not need surgery, radiation therapy and spending a lot of money, just eat properly, they can still beat cancer that modern medicine is still helpless if the disease is discovered late.

***

This book presents a few parts scientific bases such as the body's metabolism, which produces energy and protein synthesis. This process helps the body to function and with cancer patients, it also helps the cancer tumor to grow. The book also presents the causes of cancer, the harmful effects of free radicals and the harmful effects of overeating meat, especially red meat.

The author also wrote 5 stories about cancer patients who were cured by the vegetarian diet. They are extraordinary stories but completely true.

The author hopes people read and apply those healing experiences when needed. If having determination and understanding, the patient will beat cancer.

Ho Chi Minh City, Viet Nam

February 1, 2020

**DONG LA**

# PART I: 5 EXTRAORDINARY STORIES BUT TRUE IN THE FIGHT AGAINST CANCER

## Story Nº 1: The writer who used to be a pharmaceutical chemical researcher has cured himself and helped his friend cure cancer

I studied Chemistry at the University of Ho Chi Minh City. After graduating, I was invited to work at a pharmaceutical research institute. It is the Institute of Pharmaceutical Industry under the Ministry of Health of Vietnam. At this research institute, my first project was joining a team of researchers extracting Berberine, an active ingredient found in Coscinium usitatum. This plant grows many in the forest of Vietnam. Berberine is an alkaloid used to treat diarrhea, dysentery, intestinal inflammation, jaundice, fever, malaria, poor digestion, and eye pain.

Then, I participated in some other projects, but the most memorable was that I was assigned to lead a team to extract the vinblastine, an anticancer active substance in Catharanthus roseus (Vinca rose). This plant grows wild and is grown as an ornamental plant. Vinblastin is used to treat leukemia (cancer of the white blood cells). The vinblastine content in Vinca roses is very low, only about 1 in 10,000. From 10 tons of Vinca roses (dried) can only extract 1 kg of vinblastine. Therefore, the work is very difficult. We extracted the active ingredients with Ethanol ($C_2H_5OH$), and then isolated Vinblastine with a system of chromatographic columns. Vinblastine has a very high price, millions of dollars per kilogram. With the laboratory scale, we extracted a few grams. I was very happy to prepare for the project on a larger scale.

But then, a thing unexpectedly happened. I, the head of the research team, was replaced because the new director of the research institute did not like me. The former director who liked me was retired. I was not surprised because I knew there was a confrontation between the leaders of the institute.

I was saddened to suddenly not be able to continue the project that was not completed. I felt like a mother whose baby was jerked off her arm. After I left, the conflict at the institute continued for some years, and then the institute finally disintegrated; and of course, my cancer research project has never been completed.

Then I applied for a job at the Agricultural Chemical Research Center of Vietnam Pesticides Company. Here I was again assigned to lead a team and continuing to research and to produce a pest control product that preserves postharvest agricultural products. This project had lasted for more than 20 years but had never been completed because the active ingredient of that product causes fire and explosions. After three years, I finished that work. An International Workshop (hosted by ACCT and Bordeaux) on Reducing Postharvest Loss, with 18 participating countries, tested my product in Binh Tay rice warehouse. It was evaluated to be equivalent to a German product. A member of the French delegation asked to buy our products for use in France. Then my research work was sent to the contest "Creating about Science and Technology" of Ho Chi Minh City 1993 and I was awarded A which was the highest award.

And, the strange fate led me, a person working in pharmaco-chemical research, to meet the top literary talents in Vietnam including the great poet Che Lan Vien. I wrote poetry, prose, reasoning, and criticism, and became a member of the Vietnam Writers Association. I have many memories with Che Lan Vien, especially the story that he had lung cancer, had surgery at Cho Ray Hospital, but in the end, he failed to pass.

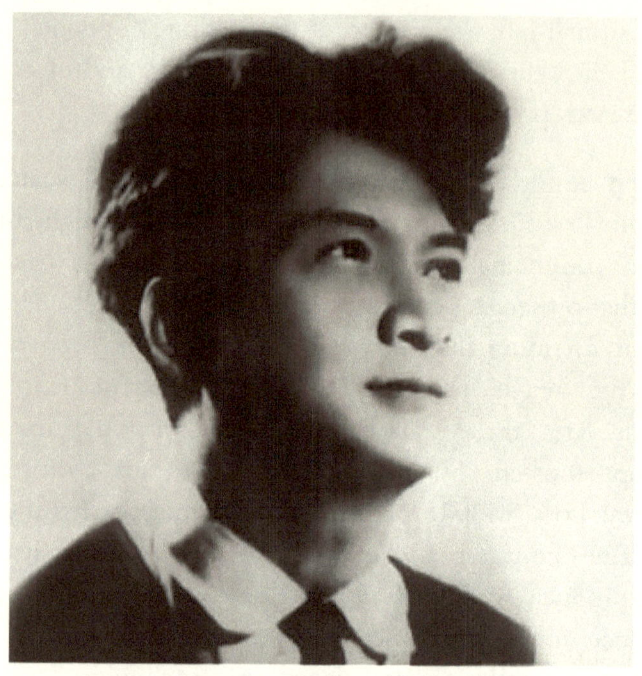

The poet Che Lan Vien

Source: http://phunuonline.com.vn/van-hoa-giai-tri/chuyen-tinh-danh-nhan/che-lan-vien-1920-1989-cat-dut-long-anh-trang-cua-em-100785/

***

More than ten years ago, the friend, who lived in the same village as me ago, had a wife with brain cancer. I went to bookstores to find buying a book that could help me learn about cancer treatments to help them. I bought a book written about an eating way to cure cancer of George Oshawa. It is the "Macrobiotic" diet that is primarily vegetarian, a simple method but difficult to practice. In order to change from a normal diet to a vegetarian diet, we must overcome habits and appetites.

More active in curing cancer, the book also provides evidence of fasting patients during the time they can bear to starve and destroy cancerous tumors. If we fast, surely we will be very hungry and uncomfortable. Therefore, it is required to have a very high level of knowledge and determination to be able to perform the hunger strike for healing.

I was very happy bringing the book I bought to the friend whose wife had cancer. Unfortunately, this couple was unable to understand the deep meaning of the book. Their area of specialization was the social field, so they could not understand about science and medicine. The husband still to give his wife eating a lot of meat and fish in the meals, did the opposite to the healing base of the book. I could not stop him because he loved his wife very much.

As a result, as the tumor grew in the brain and made the wife lose gradually her consciousness, and eventually, it killed her.

***

There was a similar story; my wife's family also has a sad story. Her uncle is a priest and the head of a church. He also had liver cancer, after years of hepatitis B virus infection.

I also gave him the book writing about cancer treatment by the vegetarian diet and I used my ability to explain science to a priest who specializes in preaching. He listened to me, ate vegetarian food for about a month. So glad when he went to the hospital for the examination, the doctor announced that his liver enzymes were reduced. But some Sueur, who had too much love for their priest, went to buy some "ac" chickens, a kind of chicken whose meat is black, commonly used for Chinese medicine to nourish the sick. They cooked that "ga ac" meat to him eating. In this case, the word "ac" means both "black" and "evil", it was right "evil". That meat was not good for the sick, but it was good for the tumor, nourishing the tumor to grow. After eating, my wife's uncle was taken to the hospital for emergency treatment and he died a few days later.

***

And then, I, the author of this book, about 7 years ago, I saw the mole under my left eye suddenly becoming very itchy and fast-growing. I suspect it transforming into melanoma. I remembered the vegetarianism against cancer written in the book I bought for the friend had the wife with brain cancer and thought, "It's time I must apply it myself."

I thought tumor cells grow faster than normal cells so they needed more nutrients. They also need nutrients to "build" the tumor just like people need materials to build a home. The material main is the amino acids that are created after the digestive process the protein of the food and most importantly the essential amino acids because the body cannot synthesize itself.

Therefore, I decided not to eat anything just drink coconut water. I feel normal health, but the body is empty and hungry feeling is really terrible. However, knowing melanoma was dangerous cancer, I was determined to do it. Between hunger and death, I had to choose one of the two and I chose hunger.

After about 10 days, I asked my nephew: "How did my mole change?" He replied: "I saw the edge of it being exfoliated."

I was happy to find that drinking coconut water was effective so, but I was still worried, "Is my mole really cancer?" I was more determined. After I continued to drink coconut water for a few more days, finally, the dangerous mole dropped itself. How aghast! I believe it is a melanoma. At my neck, there's a big mole that is still intact. Because it is a normal mole, it is not affected by my eating!

A small thing, but it is proof of a great and wonderful scientific problem.

Cancer patients can change their diet to cut off the tumor's supply of nutrients so that it will die and they will recover.

***

And a few months before the first time I went to America, a friend had an appointment with me after he had surgery to remove liver cancer. I went to see my friend and the next part of this book will be our story.

# Story Nº 2: Seeing the friend with liver cancer

Before the Lunar New Year, a friend in Nha Trang city, named Nguyen Khac Ke, called me:

"Mr. Hung (my real name), after the Lunar New Year, I will go to Cho Ray Hospital for re-examination, I like to see you again! I am very sick so I cannot talk for a long time now. When we meet, we will talk more."

Although the friend did not say clearly, I still felt something was very bad. Later on February 16 (solar calendar), we met each other. He told me that he had to come to the hospital for tests because he had surgery for liver cancer!

***

Cho Ray Hospital, which my friend said is the place with many unforgettable impressions in my life.

In 1989, Che Lan Vien, a great poet in Vietnam, whom I considered as my father, had lung cancer. The doctors operated for him at Cho Ray Hospital.

That day, I witnessed the moment that the nurses pushed the stretcher to bring him out of the operating room. His face was swollen. He had a lung operation so it was very hard to breathe. His body was covered with a white cloth.

Later, he recovered very quickly, as if nothing had happened. However, the cancer cells, remaining after surgery, developed rapidly, metastasized to his brain. He gradually lost consciousness and finally, he was dead!

The wife, whose husband lived in the same village as me, with brain cancer, also had surgery in the Cho Ray Hospital. I still vividly remembered that day. I also saw some nurses pushing the stretcher to bring her out of the operating room to her room. In the same room with her, there was a girl who had been operated earlier. It seems the anesthetic ran out, she is moaning painfully. After that, my friend's wife quickly recovered. Just like Che Lan Vien, the cancer cells remaining after surgery developed rapidly into a large tumor in her brain, causing her to lose gradually consciousness, and finally, she also died.

Now, the friend in Nha Trang also has liver cancer due to the Hepatitis B virus. Unfortunately for most cancer patients in Vietnam, when the disease discovered is usually late, It was more like a death sentence to them.

For example, singer Trần Lập recently still sang on television, and singer Minh Thuận recently also played on the "familiar faces" program, now both of them died of cancer.

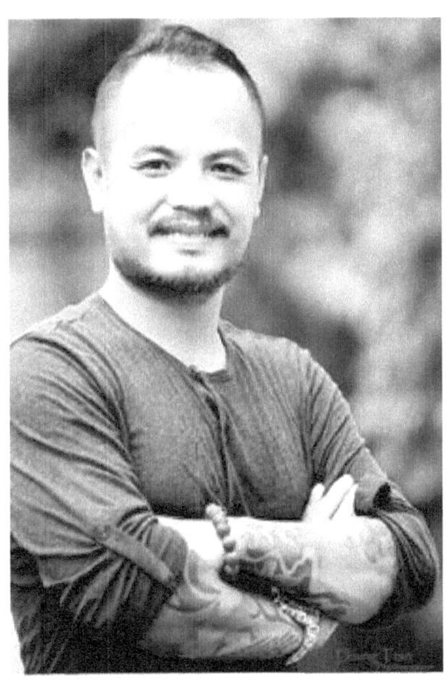

Singer Tran Lap

When it comes to cancer treatment, the surgeons often opt for the surgical procedure to remove the tumor, followed by chemotherapy and radiotherapy. The success rate of surgical procedure in the remove of the tumor can only be high if the disease was detected early and the tumors are small. The doctors are able to remove whole tumors, no cancer cells remain, and the patient will be cured. But if the disease discovered was late and the tumor has grown, although the doctors cut it off, the remaining cancer cells still would grow and spread to other parts of the body, forming new tumors. Therefore, after surgery, doctors usually perform chemotherapy and radiation. However, these therapies not only kill cancer cells but also destroy healthy cells in the bone marrow, stomach and intestines, and can damage organs such as the liver, kidneys, heart, brain, and lungs. Chemotherapy and radiation usually reduce the size of the tumor at its initial stages.  The long-term use will not destroy the tumor anymore, causing the immune system to be damaged or destroyed, so the body will not be able to withstand infections and complications. Chemotherapy and radiation can also cause cancer cells to mutate and become resistant and difficult to kill. So, when the cancer is discovered late, the tumor has grown up, it's like the boxer still "knock out" modern medicine.

Before going to Cho Ray Hospital to meet my friend who had surgery for liver cancer, I went to look for the book about George Oshawa's Macrobiotic eating method. I copied it to make some new books. I want to give a book to my friend and the rest will be given to someone in need.

***

Afternoon 16-2, my friend phoned:

"Mr. Hung, I have been checked. You come to Cho Ray Hospital, please. When you come, phone me, I will go out to see you."

I went to the hospital. After a few years, we meet again, I see my friend changed a lot. He is five years younger than me but looks a lot older. His face looks pale and gray. His hair and beard are white. However, he is still cheerful and not pessimistic.

I took him to a cafe nearby. We went inside and after ordered two cups of coffee, I asked:

"Now, you say your treatment "strategy". I will give you some suggestions."

"I'm generally vegetarian and meditating."

"That's the right direction, but the most important thing is whether you can maintain a vegetarian diet. You have to overcome yourself, have to beat the eating habits, and have to beat the greediness. People often say, "Saying very easily, but doing very difficulty." In short, you have to be completely vegetarian."

The TET just passed, the meal was full of fish and meat, but I only ate vegetables, bulbs, and fruits, and I just drank some milk to get protein."

At this point, I gave him the book and said:

"You drink milk is wrong! Now, I give you this book. First, you read the story of a doctor, the director of a hospital in the United States. He has cancer. When he was pushed to the wall foot, he was forced to adopt the Japanese vegetarianism diet to treat cancer. He kept disciplined, still working, meeting and partying, but he always carried a box of vegetarian food to eat alone.

There are many ways to explain the mechanism of cancer treatment by vegetarianism. I see the tumor as a plant sprout, so it grows stronger than the normal cells of the body. Therefore, it needs nutrition many times more than the body's normal requirements. Its main nutrition is amino acids, the materials for cancer tumor cells to multiply. If you cut off the source of the nutrient supply to it, it will die. This explains the cases in which a cancer patient practices a "hunger strike" that will cause the cancer tumor to die before the body. There was a woman who had a tumor in her nostrils. She went on a hunger strike for some time that she could tolerate, and eventually, the tumor fell out.

I myself had a mole under my left eye. It suddenly gets very itchy and grows fast. I suspected it turned into melanoma which is a type of cancer. I decided not to eat anything and just drank coconut water. After more than 10 days, the mole also fell out.

According to physiology, the human body only stores fat to provide energy when needed, not stores proteins to provide amino acids. People who eat a lot of fat, sugar, and starch will certainly get fat, but if they eat a lot of meat, the excess will be excreted and the muscles will not grow. Only the muscles of children and those who exercise especially bodybuilding will grow. The protein synthesis of both normal cells and tumors needs the supply of amino acids from the digestion of food.

In the case of vegetarians who eat plant protein instead of animal protein can cure cancer because plant protein is the protein containing low levels of essential amino acids. Lack of any essential amino acid both normal and cancer cells in the body will not synthesize the protein. If you eat a variety of plant proteins, your body still has enough essential amino acids to function and survive, but they are not redundant for the tumor.

Both the body and the tumor need glucose to provide energy, which is like the gasoline needed for cars, and the amino acids needed to synthesize proteins that are like bricks needed for building houses. Therefore, in order to treat cancer more positively, in my opinion, cancer patients need to fast for the time they can tolerate, then eat vegetable protein instead of meat, the treatment result will definitely be better. Long enough fasting is an important factor in killing tumors, but weak and lean people cannot practice it. We need to understand that fasting is for healing, not fasting for death. Therefore, it is necessary to perform the fast gradually, many times and the time of fasting is long or short depending on the patient's body condition.

On the contrary, meat and fish contain a higher percentage of essential amino acids than vegetable protein. In daily meals, people often eat more animal protein than the body needs. This will cause an excess of amino acids in general and especially essential amino acids, and main this excess are the source of nutrients for the growth of tumors. Therefore, in short, you have to eat completely vegetarian."

"Ok, I will also eliminate milk. I bought it at the hospital canteen. They sold it to foster the patient. I will bring the bottles of milk bought to go home for my wife and children to drink."

Finished speaking, he took the cigarettes in his bag to invite me. I shook my head. He lit a cigarette then asked:

"You have quit smoking, right? I also quit smoking but sometimes I still smoke."

"You smoke so is wrong! You should remember that you are facing death. I'm a writer so I want to say so impressively that, if you die also as a rat die, a cockroach dies. Now you have to quit immediately. Smoking not only causes lung cancer but also the toxins and the free radicals will enter the bloodstream. For healthy people, they may not be affected much, but to you, the cells were and still are transforming into cancer, so these cells just need to be slightly stimulated that they will develop."

"Ok, I will also quit smoking completely!"

I thought I said all that I needed to say to a friend who was carrying a serious illness, so I left. But I know it is difficult for my friend to achieve his goal. People do not easily give up eating or living habits, even knowing very well that these habits are harmful to their health.

Like the story I told, I only drink coconut water when the moles under my left eye suddenly itched and developed abnormally. As I wrote, it was terrible to be hungry, but between hunger and death, I had to choose one of the two, and I chose the hunger. Finally, the mole was fallen out!

***

My friend came back to Nha Trang. He followed carefully my instructions. Three months after surgery, when he returned to the hospital for a checkup, the doctor found no cancerous tumor. Around the same time, when he was infected with the hepatitis B virus and was not a vegetarian yet, from liver status nothing, the doctor said he had four liver tumors!

He also shared on Facebook an interesting story such as confirming what I advised him, should be vegetarian to fight cancer, is right.

He wrote that he had a friend had Lung cancer. This man had a malignant lump as big as a teacup in his lungs. Sadly, the doctors were helpless, told him to go home and wait for death. The tumor could not be cut because it was close to the aorta. He went back home and started his own therapy through avoiding sugar, meat, fish and rice in the meals, and just drinking mixture water of vegetables, carrots, radishes, beetroot, oranges, and apples. After three months, the tumor decreased its size a lot and after nine months, the cancerous tumor completely disappeared. Now he is healthy, working and eating normally again. Four people with cancer like him had been treated by chemotherapy and radiotherapy, at last, all four people died.

***

And finally, I was very happy because I saw the friend in Nha Trang who had liver cancer posted on Facebook:

"For the first nine months of treatment, the AFP index was 6.8

below the normal range of 10. I'm so happy so I reward myself with two 333 cans of beer. "

I wrote about this story and posted it on my blog, sometimes thousands of US readers read that post at the same time.

***

That was the story that happened three years ago.

Recently, VietNam.Net has posted continuously some information that oncologists opposed a vegetarian diet to treat cancer after they have emergency cases of critical malnutrition due to vegetarianism.

In my opinion, the vegetarian diet to cure cancer is not simple; vegetarians need to understand in order to perform properly, and must have a very high determination to maintain.

People who don't know, be a vegetarian like a believer leading to severe malnutrition, is false; Besides, cancer doctors have made themselves standard, not understanding about vegetarianism, anti-vegetarian is also wrong!

After I wrote the book again, I wondered, "what if I also think wrongly?" As for my friend Ke, there was a problem. Because of a trifling thing Ke was sulky and cut off contact with me, 3 years have passed, do not know still to live or died? Ke is not only a friend but also a witness to my explanation of the ability of a vegetarian diet to cure cancer. If Ke did as I said and still did not survive, I was wrong.

The wrong speech was bad; writing books that spread the wrong around the world is worse and causes great harm. Therefore, yesterday I called Ke, thinking, "If He's not alive, it's true that I'm calling a ghost." Happy to have the bell, and happier to see Ke's voice:

"Hello, who are you?" (Meaning deleted my number)

"I'm glad to hear your voice."

"Well... Mr. Hung?"

"It's funny! What did you sulk to do for? It is your health that is important. How are you now?"

Ke said that he was still completely vegetarian, his liver tumor did not recur, and it was true that there was a mysterious predestination to set us up to meet again, after two years of non-contact, when I call "a lo", Ke answered, " I'm in Sài Gòn ". Yesterday afternoon, which was immediately after my call, Ke told his son to drive him immediately to my house.

Seeing Ke again, I was very happy and happier when Ke affirmed that being a vegetarian has the effect of curing cancer, if not a vegetarian, "died a long time ago!" However, I deeply sympathize with Ke.  Ke was 4 years younger than me, but because of illness, Ke looked much older and weaker than me.

I told my daughter to take pictures of me and Ke as a living witness who defeated cancer.

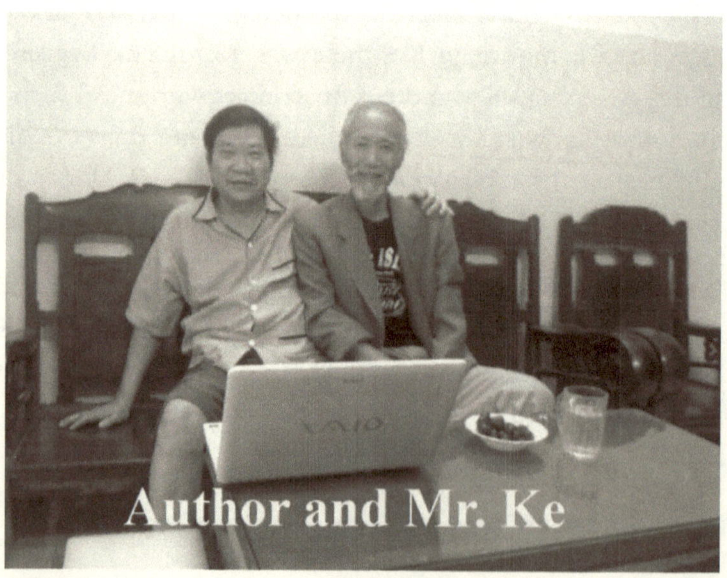

When I wrote the meeting between me and Ke and posted the article and the photo on Facebook, Ke commented, "After surgery, people usually ate many kinds of nutritious food, but after I had surgery, I went home and transferred to a 100% vegetarian diet. Thanks to that, after 3 years of surgery, the condition of the liver is normal, many indicators are sometimes better than people without cancer. Every 3 months to come to Cho Ray to re-examine, only to receive a sentence from BS: "Your liver is normal, go home and come back for 3 months later!!!!!"

# The story N°3: The doctor, a director of a hospital in the US that eats vegetarian food to cure cancer

In the book, Vegetarianism To Prevent and Cure Cancer, which I gave my friend, had a story about Dr. Anthony Sattinaro, director of a large hospital in Philadelphia (USA). He had testicular cancer, prostate cancer (grade IV) and rib cancer. In three weeks he had to go to the operating table three times, cut off testicle, prostate, and finish with an examination of bone. According to modern medicine, he will have been able only more to live a short time. But then, by chance, he changed his eating habits, ate vegetarian food instead of ordinary food. At last, he was cured of the disease.

He wrote his story and it was published in Paris Match Magazine 10-1982 (France); Life Magazine 8-1982 (USA); Journal of Atarashiki Sekaia 10-1982 (Japan), and Newspaper "Đại đoàn kết" 11-1988 (Vietnam).

Anthony Sattinaro has a father who lives in Long Beach. His father had just died of cancer. Attending the funeral finished, he drove back to Philadelphia. On the way, he met two young men with long hair covering their ears. They begged him to let them to go with him.

The story had Eastern spirituality color because he often hate young men with such long hair, but did not know why he let them go with him this time, and later he thought that the two guys had a "mission" to save him. He stopped for two young men to enter the car, and then continued the journey. They started talking to each other. Two guys told him that they had graduated from a cooking class, and he also did not hide his sadness. He told them that he had just buried his father died of cancer and that he also was dying of cancer.

He was surprised by the attitude of the two young men when they heard his very bad news as if nothing was important. One of the two told him, "You do not have to die. Cancer is not difficult to cure. You just need to change your eating habits; you need have to completely eliminate the meat and fish in the meals, which means you have to completely vegetarian. "A doctor, director of a hospital in the United States, where has the most developed medical science, first heard this from the mouth of a boy, he could not believe it.

However, when he got home, he received a book about the ability of the cure for cancer by the method "macrobiotic" from those two young men. And then, there is no other way, overcome the doubts of himself and his colleagues in the hospital, he found the place of Denny Waxman, an OHSAWA method promoter in Philadelphia. However, he still cannot help thinking that he had entrusted his life to a group of quack!

Because he had Stage 4 cancer, in his meal, the Waxman family completely eliminates some of his favorite foods such as meat, milk, and processed starches, etc. He only ate 50-60% of cereals, 25% of vegetables, 15% of beans and seaweed; the rest is miso and spices. After a few weeks, he wrote: "The play in theater begins". One morning, he reached over to take the painkillers, and he was surprised to realize he had no pain anymore, "It's like having someone help me take off my shirt that is too tight". And then after the more 13 months of a vegetarian diet, he was completely cured!

***

In the view of Western medicine, the menu of Dr. Anthony Sattinaro as described above not only would fail to cure cancer but it would also mean that Dr. Anthony would die as a result of the lack of proteins in his meals.

Cellular ribosomes require different amino acids for protein synthesis. A deficiency of any amino acid will result in the protein being unable to form.

Among amino acids, about 8 amino acids that the human body completely did not synthesize are called essential amino acids. They are provided by the food we eat. If your diet lacks one of these eight important nutrients, it can lead to some serious illness. Meanwhile, from the standpoint of Western medicine, plant proteins often contain little of those essential amino acids.

However, in fact, vegetarians are not only healthy but are also cured of many diseases, including cancer.

Plant proteins are found in raw starch (brown rice) and vegetables. Children at the highest development stage need mother's milk containing 5% protein. If plant foods are compared to breast milk, we will see that rice contains 8% protein, corn has 11%, oatmeal has 15%, and bean has 27%. As such, protein deficiency is unlikely to occur if adults eat vegetables and unprocessed cereals. Therefore, the vegetarian advocates claim that the American Heart Association (AHA) statement is often quoted, "but incorrect." The statement wrote that in the plant proteins "most of them lack one. Or many essential amino acids and are, therefore, considered incomplete proteins. "

In 1952, William Rose and his colleagues identified human requirements for eight essential amino acids, giving the "minimum amino acid requirements" of a body and then doubling as considered an "absolutely safe dose". By calculating a number of essential amino acids supplied by the raw starch and comparing these values with the amounts of substances identified by Rose, the results show that any combination of the plant foods provided Amino acids all exceed the recommended requirement.

Therefore, as a paradox, the main cause of the diseases of modern times is mainly as a result of the development. For those who have a rich and leisurely life, they little work, and the more they eat, the fatter they become.

Nutrition exceeds the human's body needs will not metabolize completely. They accumulate and cause many illnesses, such as excess fat causing obesity, excess sugar causing diabetes, excess protein causing gout, and more dangerous, they create a lot of toxic substances that cause all Diseases, including cardiovascular disease and cancer.

***

If people eat red meat that rich iron ion, it will cause toxic, opposite, if people completely eat vegetarian food, they will be anemia due to iron deficiency. Therefore, researchers recommended that vegetarians could avoid anemia due to iron deficiency by eating more fruits and vegetables that are high in vitamin C.

Vitamin C increases the absorption of iron and able to against inhibition of iron absorption of phytic acid, oxalic acid, and tannic acid.

Pregnant women, breastfeeding mothers, infants, teenagers, athletes or people with much blood loss should use iron supplements. Vitamin B12 deficiency can also occur in absolute vegetarians because of plant foods that lack vitamin B12. This vitamin is recommended for pregnant women who are vegetarians. The same applies to breastfeed women and especially the elderly (The body of the elderly often little absorbs vitamin B12.) Zinc deficiency can also occur in vegetarians.

Zinc in plant foods also is little absorbed by the inhibition of phytic acid, oxalate, fiber and soy protein, and the elderly are at risk for zinc deficiency despite being vegetarian or not, so they should take tablets containing zinc.

When cooking those who eat brown rice should pay attention to plant seeds that have a self-defense mechanism by inhibiting germination to germinate in appropriate seasons. They use two active substances, abscisic acid, and phytic acid, found in bran. These two substances are harmful to health. Therefore, scientists advised us to "turn on the switch" for brown rice germination by immersing it, but only at the "germination" stage.

At this time, the poisonous ingredient inside the seed has been changed to be safe for human consumption. Then the enzymes that sleep in the rice grains at this state are stimulated to function and provide maximum nutrients.

Vegetarianism also recommends people eating the full foods that nature gives to humans, such as bran, cereals, bulbs, and roots of vegetables; need to eat raw food whenever possible to preserve vitamins and active ingredients. Tomatoes and carrots should be cooked with some oil to dissolve lycopene and carotene.

***

Vegetables, bulbs, and fruits have the effect of preventing and fighting cancer because they contain vitamins and active substances with resistance to mutations, against oxidants, inhibit cancer disease onset and isolate cancer cells to against the spread of the disease.

Vitamin C dissolved in water should strongly destroy the radicals dissolved in the water phase; Vitamin E dissolved in oil will collect and destroy free radicals in the lipids. Carotenoids are a "drink" of free oxygen, 20 times more potent than vitamin E.

Crushed eggplant and crushed spinach have the strongest effect against mutations. Crushed amaranth killed cancer cells, particularly breast cancer, liver cancer, and lung cancer. Red beetroot is considered one of the most effective vegetables for treating leukemia and cancer in general because it contains Betaine that has strong anti-cancer properties, is also a potent anti-inflammatory and anti-oxidant.

Rudolf Breuss, an Austrian researcher, used fruit juice: Beetroot (55%), carrots (20%), celery (20%), potatoes (3%), white cabbage (2%) and gave his patients drink every day. He helped more than

45,000 people with cancer and other incurable diseases to treat the disease effectively. Patients taking that juice mixture for 42 consecutive days showed that their cancer cells were completely destroyed (http://www.baomoi.com/).

## Story Nº4: The man who fasted and ate vegetarian food won the battle against cancer

In fact, many witnesses have shown that vegetarian diets can cure cancer. Why modern medicine has not studied and applied it?

Therefore, I would like to continue to tell the story of a former employee at 108 Military Hospital who had cancer. He studied the "macrobiotic" vegetarian diet and cured himself of illness.

That is Nguyen Minh Tuan (72 years old), a former employee of Military Hospital 108. His father was a doctor and the director of that hospital in the 1960s of the last century. He told that, since 1983, doctors told him that he had cancer in the final stage. Two tumors in his lungs developed large.

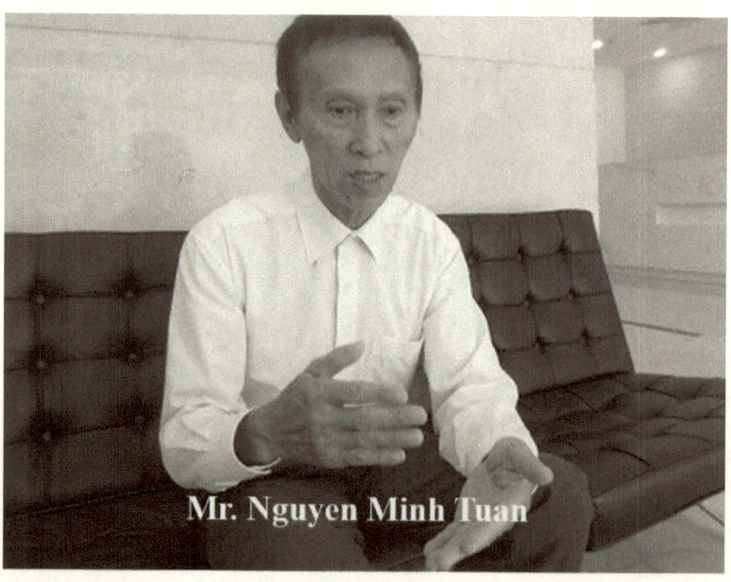


Working at Hospital 108, he had all the conditions for treatment. However, the head of the Oriental Medicine Department at the hospital showed him how to treat cancer with the method of "hunger-strike" and Macrobiotic vegetarianism of Oshawa. At the time, he had only very few documents, but he said he did not understand why he had a strong belief in that method and he decided to apply it. However, there were many people stopping him. Even until now, still many nutritional experts believe that cancer cure by fasting, eating brown rice and sesame salt is a scam and unscientific, that time, more than 30 years ago, whether could anyone agree with him? Despite the counsel, he still resolutely left the hospital, coming home to cure himself. That was August 20, 1983. The papers indicated he had cancerous tumors in the right lobes.

His father was the director of 108 Military Hospital. When he was sick, of course, his father advised him to apply Western medicine's cancer treatment. However, when he presented his ideas, his father respected that choice, but his father still does not believe it.

He ate 100% brown rice and sesame salt and only ate two meals a day, morning and afternoon, with no dinner. On Sundays, he did not eat at all. After 4 months, he had lost 25 kgs in weights. Seeing his health deteriorate, his hospital colleagues must come to his home, forcing him to go to the hospital. He was forced to obey orders. But in the hospital, he decided not to take a pill, refuse biopsy test. He only allowed doctors to radiology his lungs.

Results X-rays showed that the previous tumor, liked a chicken egg in the lungs, had disappeared altogether. The doctors were surprised. His father went to the hospital to watch X-ray films and was also shocked. Although very happy that his son had escaped death, his father remained silent. Everyone was happy, only he understood that the result is only like cutting a top of a tree; the residual disease is like the roots which are more really scary.

He explained why he had firmly decided to apply the method of "hunger-strike" and the "Macrobiotic". According to him, understanding this method was very simple. Like a tree not watered, not fertilized, its leaves would not be green. Similarly, with an animal, if it was not fed, it would be stunted and could not grow. For cancerous tumors in the human body were similar. No one can live without food or drinks. From that simple principle, we can understand that if the disease is not nourished it will also die. All plants, animals, and diseases will die when they are not provided with nutrition.

If we proceed to cleanse the blood and provide a good amount of vegetable protein to the body, it will keep the blood and the body in good condition. Eating brown rice and sesame salt is good for that. After a person fasted for a suitable amount of time, his blood would change. At this time, the human body is a clean environment, so bacteria and tumors have no nutrients to live on.

He thought everyone could apply this method, but like Western medicine treatment, vegetarianism must be started early to bring efficiency. If the patient's illness was too severe, it could not be effective.

Before "hunger-strike", it is necessary had to wash the intestines with eating diluted porridge.  On the first day, he ate three bowls of porridge in place of each meal.  2nd day halved the amount of porridge compared to the first day, the third day, ate the porridge even diluted more. The patients must ensure that nothing was left in the colon before starting "hunger-strike". In the first three days, they should eat more than 50 grams of sesame per day to increase laxative. After, they did not eat any kind of food during the process of "hunger-strike," except filtered water. When doing "hunger-strike" to the maximum threshold, the patient cannot bear more; they might eat back, started to drink from the water of brown rice roasted, and finally, ate rice.

When people use a "hunger strike" as a tool to fight cancer, whether the patient will starve to death before dying from cancer or not?  He said that people died of hunger only when there were no nutrients in the body. In this case, the "hunger-strike" was controlled; of course, it depended on whether a person was fat or skinny to determine the appropriate length of time for a hunger strike. The special thing that he reminded patients undergoing a "hunger strike" was that when eating back, they had to chew the food very carefully. Chewing like that not just helped them to swallow easily; it is also an activity that helped stimulates salivation for nutrition to be absorbed into the stomach wall in the most effective way, providing enough nutrition for the body.

Now, after 30 years of implementation "Macrobiotic" method to cure cancer, he still occasionally eats meat and fish, but only eats a small portion, and eat 1-2 times a week.

He regretted that until now, this method had not been studied in detail in Vietnam although it had helped a lot of people get cured. In 2007, the Vietnam Union of Science and Technology Associations helped a workshop on nutrition. He was invited to present at this workshop. There were many people in the workshop who said that his story was a scam, but there are also some who said that it needed to be studied in detail, based on specific information and evidence about people who had been cured of cancer, through the medical records that he together with a doctor at the Children's hospital brought to the workshop.

Scientists opposed vegetarianism because they did not understand it. He had clearly explained its scientific basis, and give the proof, some scientists had also analyzed the nutritional content of brown rice. Specifically, brown rice bran contained 120 antioxidants such as CoQ10, alpha-lipoic acid, oligomeric proanthocyanidins, SOD, tocopherol and tocotrienol, IP6 (inositol hexaphosphate), glutathione, carotenoids, selenium, phytosterols, lutein, and lycopene.

Therefore, brown rice has excellent effects in protecting the body against free radicals, supporting cancer treatment. IP6 contained in brown rice is a substance that has powerful anti-cancer activity, especially against cancer cells in the liver and intestines. With sesame salt, sesame contains large amounts of calcium, iron, and other nutrients and is an excellent source of vegetable oil that cannot produce cholesterol.

He asserted that this is not a deceptive or unscientific method as people think. However, to successfully treat cancer, patients should have the determination and very much perseverance.

The story was written by Pham Thi Ngoc Tram in her book Phương Pháp Ăn Uống Để Phòng Chống Bệnh Ung Thư (Diet to Preventing and Fighting Cancer), and the interview with Mr. Nguyen Minh Tuan of Nhat Thu - Mac Phi was posted on the newspaper Pháp Luật.online. (https://baophapluat.vn/thuoc/het-benh-cuu-can-bo-vien-108-miet-mai-nghien-cuu-ve-thuc-duong-306512.html

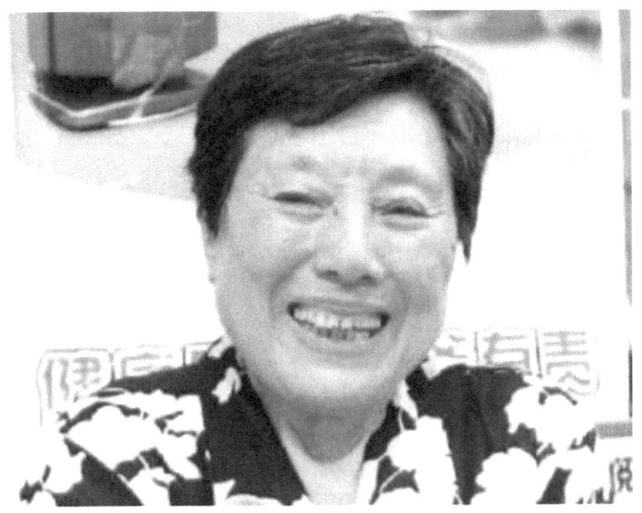

Mrs. Liu Songhan

On VN.net recently posted the post "44 years of fighting cancer and 3 metastases, the old women shared the golden secret"

At age 93, the old woman drew four habits, applied every day that can prevent cancer cells from growing.

Mrs. Liu Songhan from China, now 93 years old and diagnosed with breast cancer at the age of 49. 12 years later, the tumor recurred and metastasized to the lung. Since then, Mrs. Liu has to fight two more times when cancer cells continue to metastasize to the thyroid and kidney ...

She always told people it was miraculous to fight cancer for 44 years. She not only fully recovered but also lived a long, healthy life. Mrs. Liu revealed 4 valuable experiences to fight cancer as follows:

1. Moderation exercise

Mrs. Liu often gets up early and goes to the park with her friends to practice age-appropriate nursing exercises regardless of sun or rain.

2. Doing housework

Mrs. Liu sees daily chores as light exercises in which she often cooks with healthy foods.

3. Eating a minimum of fried and baked foods that are greasy.

Besides, Mrs. Liu also ate less salt, reducing the amount of salt consumed daily during meals.

4. Eating raw grains still bran bark,

Eating raw grains that still contains the bran coating such as brown rice, barley, oats and eat lots of vegetables, tubers, and fruits.

Mrs. Liu believes that most of the causes of illness come from eating and living habits, so in order to have a body that is not sick, everyone should practice a healthy lifestyle, change mistakes in eating habits to protect yourself and your family members.

(According to An An)

Source: https://vietnamnet.vn/vn/suc-khoe/cac-loai-benh/ung-thu/cu-ba-93-tuoi-chia-se-4-thoi-quen-chong-ung-thu-vu-602312.html

# PART II: THE "MACROBIOTIC" DIET

# George Ohsawa



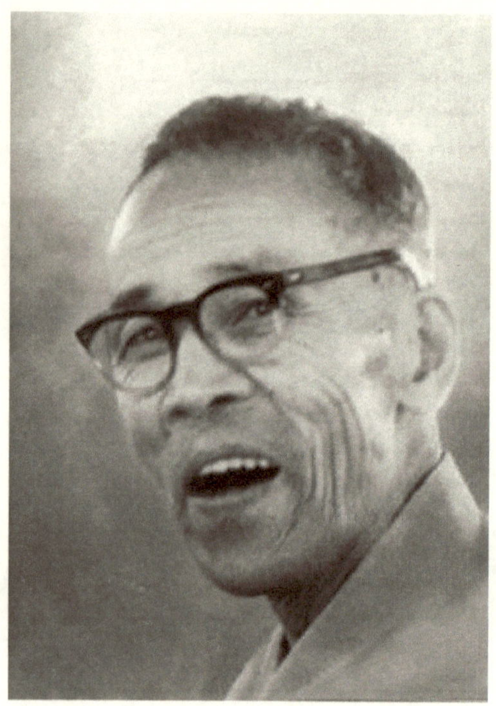

(Source: https://www.babelio.com/auteur/Georges-Ohsawa/34924)

George Ohsawa, born in Nyoichi Sakurazawa, (October 18, 1893 – April 23, 1966), was the founder of the Macrobiotic diet and philosophy. He was born in a poor samurai family in Shingu City Wakayama Prefecture, Japan.

George Ohsawa introduced the oriental principle of health to Westerners in the mid-20th century.

The gradual introduction of sugar into the Japanese diet brought in its wake the beginning of Western diseases. Dr. Sagen Ishizuka, a Japanese practitioner became famous because he cured thousands of people (through traditional use of food) after they were abandoned as incurable by the new medicine of the West.

Ohsawa states in his books that he cured himself of tuberculosis at age 19 by applying the ancient concept of yin and yang that originated in China, as well as the teachings of Sagen Ishizuka.

He traveled to Europe; particularly Paris in France where he began to spread his philosophy. After several years, he returned to Japan to start a foundation, and gather recruits for his now formalized philosophy. In 1931, he published The Unique Principle explaining the yin and yang order of the universe.

## Macrobiotic diet

A macrobiotic diet is a fad diet fixed on ideas about types of food drawn from Zen Buddhism. The diet attempts to balance the supposed yin and yang elements of food and cookware. Major principles of macrobiotic diets are to reduce animal products, eat locally grown foods that are in season, and consume meals in moderation.

A macrobiotic diet is helpful for people with cancer and other chronic diseases, although there is no good evidence to support such recommendations. Both the American Cancer Society and UK Cancer Research recommend a diet. They suggested that the macrobiotic diet improves cardiovascular disease and diabetes because it is consistent with the scientific basis of disease prevention. Macrobiotic diets are based on the concept of balancing yin and yang.

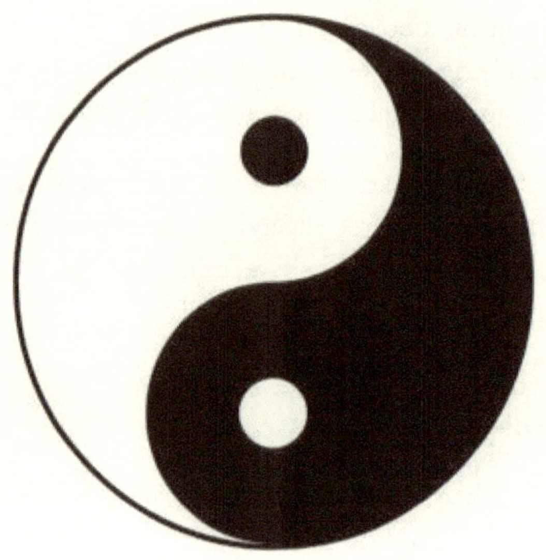



(Macrobiotic diets are based on the concept of balancing yin and yang)

Macrobiotics emphasizes locally grown whole grain cereals, pulses (legumes), vegetables, seaweed, fermented soy products, and fruit, combined into meals according to the ancient Chinese principle of balance known as yin and yang. Whole grains and whole-grain products such as brown rice and buckwheat pasta (soba), a variety of cooked and raw vegetables, beans and bean products, mild natural seasonings, fish, nuts, and seeds, mild (non-stimulating) beverages such as bancha twig tea and fruit are recommended. Some Macrobiotic proponents, including George Ohsawa, stress the fact that yin and yang are relative qualities that can only be determined in a comparison. All food is considered to have both properties, with one dominating. Foods with yang qualities are considered compact, dense, heavy, hot, whereas those with yin qualities are considered expansive, light, cold, and diffuse. However, these terms are relative; "yangness" or "yinness" is only discussed in relation to these foods to other foods.

Brown rice and other whole grains such as barley, millet, oats, quinoa, spelled, rye, and teff are considered by macrobiotics to be the foods in which yin and yang are closest to being in balance. Therefore, lists of macrobiotic foods that determine a food as yin or yang generally compare them to whole grains.

# PART III: THE SCIENTIFIC NATURE OF THE VEGETARIANISM TO CURE CANCER

# The harmful effects of eating too much animal meat

The life of each human body is maintained by physiological and biochemical processes. Physiology is all the activity of organs of the body and biochemistry is the chemical nature of these physiological activities. The end of these activities is the metabolism of nutrients to maintain the body structure, maintain the body's functioning and ultimately generate energy for all activities.

The metabolism of substances to maintain life at the same time also has side effects that cause the disease, including cancer. We all know that in addition to a small number of minerals and vitamins, the human body needs mainly water, oxygen, and nutrients. The three main nutrient groups are Lipids, Carbohydrates, and Protein.

In a textbook, an Associate Professor Ph.D. at Hanoi Medical University wrote:

"Proteins have a major role to play in the composition of all the cells, shaping the body. It is in the muscle, in the cell nucleus (the structure of DNA and RNA), in plasma (albumin, globulin, and fibrinogen). Proteins are also a major component of antibodies and enzymes in the body. Proteins have a decisive role in genetics. The genes of each individual are located on the DNA molecule that determines the genetic characteristics of the individual and the species.

The Protein of the human body is made up of 20 different amino acids, including 10 amino acids that the body does not synthesize or synthesize only a small amount compared to the needs of the body, so must be taken from the outside. They are called essential amino acids, including threonine, methionine, valine, leucine, isoleucine, lysine, arginine, phenylalanine, tryptophan, and histidine.

The Protein of each animal in the daily diet has a different amino acid ratio and differs from that of humans so it is important to have to eat a variety of protein of different animals such as fish, poultry, pork, meat cow, and milk. Vegetables and rice also have a certain ratio of protein but low protein content, so the number of protein provided is still mostly from animals. "

The above idea is not only a personal opinion but also the General theory of modern medicine. Therefore, doctors do not believe that vegetarianism can heal cancer. However, in reality, many people were healed cancer by a vegetarian diet. Their stories are still considered strange things. However, not only that, life has still more strange things. There are special cases where some people have been cured cancer with exotic and mysterious treatments that modern medicine still regards as myth and superstition.

***

This article will point out the harmful effects of the fact that people often eat too much animal meat at meals, especially for those at risk and who have had cancer. Therefore, the cancer patient should be a vegetarian, using vegetable protein instead of animal protein.

If people eat too much animal meat, especially red meat, the digestion, and the metabolism, in addition to creating nutrients nourishing the body, they can also cause the following three major damaging factors:

- Create an acid environment in the body.

- Ion Fe excess causing harm.

- Generate free radicals.

***

The ancients taught us, "knowing the enemy, knowing ourselves, fight a hundred battle, win a hundred." Therefore, we need to know the enemy of health so that we can prevent and eliminate them.

**Acidic environment**

For the body to function, nutrients such as proteins, carbohydrates, and lipids will need to be oxidized, releasing a lot of energy, some of it radiating in the form of heat, in part create substance adenosine triphosphate (ATP). It is a repository because the body only uses energy in the form of ATP.

The break of ATP's chemical bonds constantly produces energy for the body to function, converting ATP to adenosine diphosphate (ADP). ADP is quickly reverted to ATP by receiving energy from food oxidation.

Healthy people when work or exercise excessively, the sick, and the frail elderly, the blood circulation will not provide enough oxygen for cellular respiration that oxidizes nutrients (aerobic respiration), cellular respiration will be anaerobic and produces lactic acid.

Lactic acid is a substance that causes fatigue, muscle aches and, worse, an acid environment in the body.

Protein, though not the main substance, still contributes to energy supply. Protein metabolism, when the respiratory system provides oxygen deficiency, also produces lactic acid contributing to the formation of an acidic environment. In addition, when people eat too much protein, excess protein also breaks down into urea and uric acid creating an acidic environment.

In fact, many studies have shown that our health depends very much on the pH of the body. For an immune system, self-repair, and enzymes to work well, the body needs mild alkalinity at a pH of 7.35. When the body is acidic, many diseases begin to appear: allergies, osteoporosis, obesity, diabetes, migraines, gout, stroke and cancer.

Otto Heinrich Warburg, a German biologist who won the Nobel Prize in 1931, invented a theory that cancer stemming from oxygen deficiency of cell causes acidosis. In contrast, the body with high acidity also causes hypoxia. All forms of cancer are characterized by two basic conditions: acidosis and hypoxia. The nature of cancer is due to genetic mutations, perhaps the acidic environment that supports this mutation.

The metabolism of nutrients is like burning wood. If enough air, burning will be easy. In contrast, if there is a lack of air, burning will be difficult, creating smoke and leaving the wood-burning incomplete. Lactic acid and free radicals are the products of "incomplete combustion" in the body's metabolism.

**Free radical**

To date, research by scientists has shown that the main culprits of aging and disease are free radicals. In the body, they attack the cell membrane, protein molecules, and the cell nucleus, etc., causing aging and cancer.

It is estimated that each cell suffers attack about 10,000 free radicals each day. So in the life of a person who lives to 70 years of age, about 17 tons of free radicals are created.

source: https://en.wikipedia.org/wiki/Radical_(chemistry)

**Red meat and ion Fe in red meat**

University of California scientists have discovered that red meat (pork, beef, and lamb...) is detected by the human body as a foreign substance and triggers a toxic immune response. Red meat contains a sugar called Neu5Gc, when it is ingested into the stomach, causing an immune reaction, producing inflammatory antibodies and ultimately leading to cancer.

And, when red meat is under high temperatures, (such as grilled, fried,) it produces heterocyclic amino acids that also cause cancer.

Ion Fe is one of the very important minerals in the human body, especially in hemoglobin that transports oxygen in the blood to the tissues of the body. But too much iron in the diet can cause cirrhosis and liver cancer. Red meat is an iron-rich food. Iron compounds make the meat red. Iron is present in the cell as transferrin that transports proteins in plasma to the receptors on the cell surface. When transferrin is saturated with iron, it activates cell proliferation. Another iron complex is hemosiderin that is released, which may create a series of adverse effects on liver cells. Excess diet Fe also stimulates oxidation to create free radicals.

Many vegetables and fruits have antioxidant active ingredients. Vitamin C is found in many common vegetables and fruits. Some vegetables, fruits, and especially oil-rich seeds contain vitamin E. More specifically, carotene-rich carrots, lycopene-rich tomatoes, onions, and garlic contain lots of allicin, ginger contains a lot of gingerols, tea contains dissolved tannins containing catechins (EGCG), and turmeric with curcumin, etc.

Many research papers also suggest that cancer cells thrive in acidic environments. A meat-based diet creates acidic. Meat also contains antibiotics for cattle, growth hormones and parasites. All are harmful, especially to cancer patients. Instead, a diet of 80% of fresh vegetables and fruit juices, whole grains, seeds, and some fruits will bring the body back to normal alkaline environment (pH 7.35). About 20% of vegetable food can be cooked food, including beans. Fresh vegetable juice provides live enzymes that are easily absorbed and transferred to cells within 15 minutes to nourish and promote the growth of healthy cells. To have live enzymes, drink fresh vegetable juice (most vegetables including bean sprouts) and eat raw vegetables 2 or 3 times a day. Do not cook fresh vegetables because it loses many vitamins and enzymes, which are destroyed at a temperature of 104 degrees F (40 degrees C). Protein in meat is difficult to digest and requires a lot of digestive enzymes. Undigested meat lying in the intestine will rot and lead to more toxic accumulation.

Cancer cells have a hard protein shell. If you eat less meat, your body will release more enzymes to attack the protein coating of cancer cells and help the macrophage kill the cancer cells. Drinking green tea is good; it also has anti-cancer properties. It is best to use purified water to avoid the toxins and heavy metals present in tap water. Distilled water is acidic so do not drink it. Cancer is a disease of mind, body, and spirit. A dynamic life and active spirit will help cancer patients win the war against this disease and live longer.

Therefore, cancer patients need to eat vegetable protein instead of animal protein. Conversely, they need to eliminate the causes of an acidic environment, eliminate the excess of Fe ions in the diet, and eliminate the causes of free radical formation. All of these factors have the potential to prevent cancer. In addition, they need to combine with a diet rich in fruits and vegetables that contain vitamin C, vitamin E, β-carotene, polyphenols, flavonoids, selenium, etc. All of them not only nourish the body but also fight against oxidation, free radicals, aging, and disease.

# The tumor died of its greediness!

According to Vietnam Net, in a parliamentary session, an official of the National Assembly of Vietnam said, "Each year, cancer is responsible for about 70,000 deaths and over 200,000 new cases are reported to be due to unsafe food."

However, Health Minister, Associate Professor Nguyen Thi Kim Tien, said, "There are no grounds to say that many cancer patients die because of food safety."

The answer surprised many people; some people wrote articles to ridicule the knowledge of the minister. But Mrs. Tien is an Associate Professor Ph.D. of medicine, a former director of Pasteur Institute Ho Chi Minh City, head of the department at the University of Medicine and Pharmacy HCM city.

Mrs. Tien explained:

"The ministry invited experts from within and even outside the country to find out the causes of cancer deaths. The results show that the leading causes of cancer are chronic infections. For example, hepatitis B and hepatitis C which causes chronic hepatitis and liver cancer."

To those who have a deep understanding, the minister is right. The harmful effect of food poisoning is acute; the patient must be taken to the emergency room immediately for treatment. If the poisoning is too severe or the emergency is so delayed, the patient will die.

Cancer is caused by genetic mutations due to several factors such as radiation, free radicals (by metabolism), toxins (smoking, food containing pesticides, and mold), etc. They are factors that not toxic enough to kill instantly the body cells, but they are capable to mutate slowly the cell's DNA.

If the DNA was mutated, the cell will start growing out of control. It does not comply with Apoptosis (the death of cells that occurs as a normal and controlled part of an organism's growth or development) causing the formation of cancerous tumors. Mutagenic chemicals may have chemical properties that react with groups of DNA macromolecule, distort its normal action.

There is a document that shows people with hepatitis B eat moldy foods that contain aflatoxin will increase the risk of cancer 60 times higher than people only with - hepatitis B.

***

About the causes of cancer, the understanding of all people is quite consistent. On treatment, the views between orthodox medicine and unorthodox methods still have opposite opinions of each other. With cancer patients at the developmental stage, modern medicine is still powerless. In contrast, there is cancer patients using unofficial treatments were cured. The most popular and used method is George Ohsawa's vegetarian theory. However, to this day, it has not been thoroughly studied and is applied by modern medicine. Doctors still recommend that cancer patients need to eat enough protein, carbohydrates, fats, vitamins, and minerals so that the body can prevent cancer cells from growing. These are found in the main foods such as meats, vegetables, fruits, and grains.

Dr. Pham Cam Phuong, deputy director of the Center for Nuclear Medicine and Oncology, Bach Mai Hospital, also said that if the patient had cancer, no diabetes, hyperlipidemia, they should not diet. He said:

"Do not think that if you do not eat, then the tumor does not grow. This is completely wrong. The tumors are still growing. They take the substances of your body whether you eat or not. If the patients do not eat or drink, their body will be exhausted, not healthy enough to be treated with subsequent therapies to reduce the growth of the tumors and prevent them from spreading."

If according to the doctors, people with severe cancer are cured, there is nothing more to say about their views. But in reality, despite being positively treated by doctors, they still die.

The doctor at Bach Mai Hospital was wrong to say that if people did not eat, the tumor could still grow from the source of the body's own nourishment.

Johns Hopkins Hospital, Baltimore, USA, has done cancer research to answer the question: "What nourishes cancer cells?" They wrote: "Sugar is a carcinogen. Cutting of sugar is cutting off an important source of food for cancer cells." This is based on the invention of Otto Warburg, who was awarded the Nobel Prize in 1931. He found that cancer cells use energy through the fermentation of sugar.

In my opinion, the author of this book, sugar is the substance that creates the energy for the tumor acts like gasoline for the engine running. Cutting of sugar is importance; however, the cutting of material source "to build" for the tumor is more important. That is the source of protein is supplied from the food. The human body stores only fat, sugar and does not store protein. Therefore, in the body, there is no available source of nutrients that provide the material for the growth of cancerous tumors. Both the normal cells of the human and cancer cells synthesize the proteins from amino acids, especially, in which 8 essential amino acids are supplied obligatory from food because the body does not synthesize itself. Normal cells synthesize proteins for functional activities of the body, while cancer cells synthesize proteins for the growth of tumors.

In fact, there are some cases showing that if the food supply is cut, the tumor will die before the patient.

The story of a woman with a tumor in her nose fasting that caused it falling out can be an example.

And I myself also may be a witness with the story that I told about the mole under my left eye suddenly becoming itchy and fast-growing. I didn't eat any food, just drink coconut water and after about 10 days, the dangerous mole fell off itself.

There was a very rare story happening. It is proof for researchers to understand how human survival depends on nutrition?

There is a story published in some newspapers in Vietnam. In 1981, 10 Irish prisoners of the Republican Army (IRA) went on a hunger strike. Nine out of 10 men die of starvation after from 57 to 73 days (means an average of 61.6 days) when they lose about 40% of their body weight. Doctors find that while people are hungry, the body's stored protein is usually protected and for vital energy, the body mainly uses from fat reserves. It is estimated that by the time of the death, hunger strikers lose 94% of their fat, but only 19% of the protein is lost. They died because they ran out of fat, not because they ran out of protein. Therefore, this story once more proves that, if cancer patients completely cut off the protein sources in their diet, the body can still live for some time, but tumors cannot; it will die. This is the scientific basis to destroy the cancerous tumor by starving it. Of course, patients should only use the method of fasting for an appropriate time that they can tolerate and then should be vegetarian.

If a person eats vegetarian food in a scientific way, the body will have enough nutrients, not only not weak but also healthier, and can still cure cancer.

But why can people cure cancer if they eat protein from plant sources instead of protein from animal sources in vegetarian diets? It is easy to answer this question because plant protein contains a low percentage of essential amino acids. If the protein synthesis in cancer cells lacks any essential amino acids, protein macromolecules will not be formed. If there is no protein to give to the malignant tumor, it will not grow and will die.

These are the reasons that cause the tumor to die because of its greediness!

Interestingly, plant proteins contain small amounts of essential amino acids; If they are used scientifically, they will provide enough amino acids to the body, but not excess for tumors. This is the weapon that kills cancer. It's like poverty also has a good point, because it forces people eating moderation, avoid eating too much to cause diseases.

# The metabolism in the body

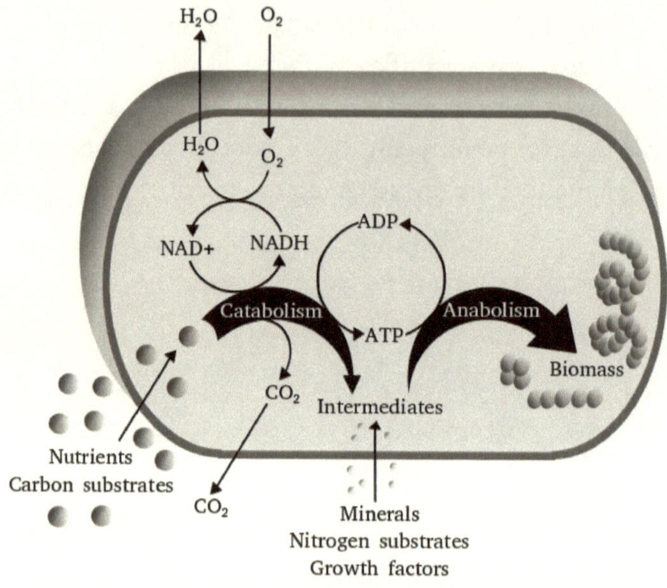



Source

https://en.wikipedia.org/wiki/Metabolism#/media/File:Metabolism.png

## Cellular metabolism

Substances formed by digestion are transported to each cell by the bloodstream. They pass through cell membranes and enter the cell interior. Once inside a cell, a compound undergoes further metabolism, usually in a series of chemical reactions. For example, a sugar molecule is broken down inside a cell into carbon dioxide and water, with the release of energy. But that process does not occur in a single step. Instead, it takes about two dozen separate chemical reactions to convert the sugar molecule to its final products.

The purpose of these reactions is to release energy stored in the sugar molecule. To explain that process, one must know that a sugar molecule consists of carbon, hydrogen, and oxygen atoms held together by means of chemical bonds. A chemical bond is a force of attraction between two atoms. That force of attraction is a form of energy. A sugar molecule with two dozen chemical bonds can be thought of as containing two dozen tiny units of energy. Each time a chemical bond is broken; a unit of energy is released.

Cells have evolved remarkable methods for capturing and storing the energy released in catabolic reactions. Those methods make use of very special chemical compounds, known as energy carriers. An example of such compounds is adenosine triphosphate generally known as ATP. ATP is formed when an adenosine diphosphate (ADP) combines with a phosphate group. The following equation represents that change:

$$ADP + P \rightarrow ATP$$

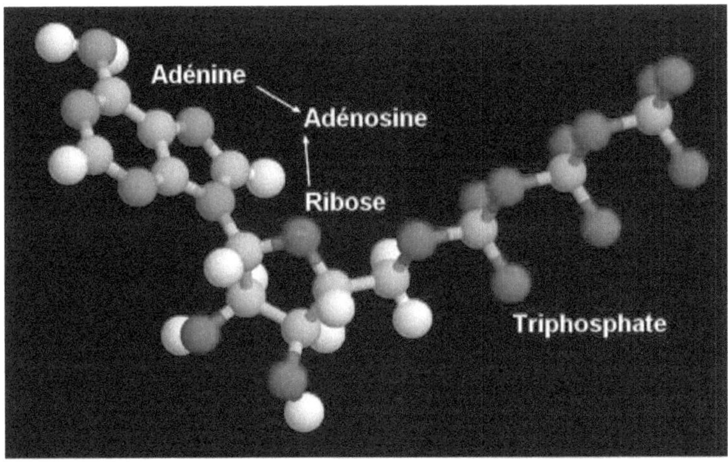


ADP will combine with a phosphate group only if energy is added to it. In cells, that energy comes from the catabolism of compounds such as sugars, glycerol, and fatty acids.

Metabolism can be divided into two categories:

Catabolism - the decomposition of molecules to store energy.

Anabolic - uses energy to synthesize all the compounds needed for cells.

The formed ATP molecule occupies the energy previously stored in the sugar molecule. Whenever a cell needs energy for a certain process, it can draw energy from an ATP molecule.

ATP is made up of three systems in muscles: the phosphate energy system, the Glycogen-Lactic acid system, and the oxygen energy system. In that with the Lactic Acid Glycogen System, muscle cells separate glycogen into glucose, no need oxygen, create ATP and lactic acid. In contrast, the oxygen system needs oxygen to oxidize sugar, protein and fat nutrients to generate energy. Oxidation of sugar as sugar hydrolysis in the lactic acid system but with oxygen; causes lactic acid to continue oxidizing to CO2 and water.

The reverse of the process shown above also takes place inside cells. That is, energy from an ATP molecule can be used to put simpler molecules together to make more complex molecules. For example, suppose that a cell needs to repair a break in its cell wall. To do so, it will need to produce new protein molecules. Those protein molecules can be made from amino acids in the metabolic pool. A protein molecule consists of hundreds or thousands of amino acid molecules joined to each other.

The energy needed to form all the new chemical bonds needed to hold the amino acid units together comes from ATP molecules.

**Metabolic disorder**

Most of the time, the metabolism works well. But sometimes a person's metabolism can cause major mayhem in the form of a metabolic disorder. In a broad sense, a metabolic disorder is any disease that is caused by an abnormal chemical reaction in the body's cells.

Most disorders of metabolism involve either abnormal levels of enzymes or hormones or problems with how those enzymes or hormones work. When the metabolism of body chemicals is blocked or defective, it can cause a buildup of toxic substances in the body or a lack of substances needed for normal body function, either of which can cause serious symptoms.

Metabolic diseases include:

## Hyperthyroidism

Hyperthyroidism is caused by an overactive thyroid gland. It causes symptoms such as weight loss, increased heart rate and blood pressure, protruding eyes, and swelling in the neck from an enlarged thyroid (goiter). The disease may be controlled with medicines or through surgery or radiation treatments.

Hypothyroidism is caused by a nonexistent or underactive thyroid gland. Untreated hypothyroidism can lead to brain and growth problems in infants and children. Hypothyroidism slows body processes and causes tiredness, slow heart rate, weight gain, and constipation. Teens who have it can be treated with oral thyroid hormone.

Metabolic diseases that are inherited are called inborn errors of metabolism. When babies were born, they were sick. Inborn errors of metabolism include galactosemia (babies born with this do not have enough of the enzyme that breaks down the sugar in milk, called galactose) and phenylketonuria (this is due to a defect in the enzyme that breaks down the amino acid phenylalanine, needed for normal growth and protein production). Inborn errors of metabolism can sometimes lead to serious problems if they're not controlled with diet or medicine from an early age.

## Type 1 diabetes

Type 1 diabetes happens when the pancreas doesn't make and secrete enough insulin. Symptoms of this disease include excessive thirst and peeing, hunger, and weight loss. Over time, the disease can cause kidney problems, pain due to nerve damage, blindness, and heart and blood vessel disease. Teens with type 1 diabetes need regular insulin injections and should control their blood sugar levels to reduce the risk of developing problems from diabetes.

## Type 2 diabetes

Type 2 diabetes happens when the body can't respond normally to insulin. Symptoms are similar to those of type 1 diabetes. Many children and teens who develop type 2 diabetes are overweight, and this is thought to play a role in their decreased responsiveness to insulin. Some teens can be treated successfully with dietary changes, exercise, and oral medicine; others will need insulin injections. Controlling blood sugar levels reduces the risk of developing the same kinds of long-term health problems that happen with type 1 diabetes.

## Digestion of food

Digestion is a necessary first step for all foods. Digestion results in the formation of smaller molecules that are able to enter a person's bloodstream. It includes simple sugars (formed by the breakdown of complex carbohydrates), glycerol and fatty acids (formed by the breakdown of lipids), and amino acids (formed by the breakdown of proteins). Cells use substances in the metabolic pool as building materials.

Metabolism is closely linked to nutrition. Essential nutrients supply energy (calories) and supply the necessary chemicals, which the body itself cannot synthesize like oxygen, nitrogen, carbon, hydrogen, sulfur, phosphorus, and around 20 other inorganic elements. The major elements are supplied in carbohydrates, lipids, and protein. In addition, vitamins, minerals, and water are necessary.

## Carbohydrate

Foods supply carbohydrates in three forms: starch, sugar, and cellulose (fiber). Body tissues depend on glucose for all activities. The overall reaction to the combustion of glucose is written as:

$$C_6H_{12}O_6 + 6\ O_2 \rightarrow 6\ CO_2 + 6\ H_2O + energy$$

Most people consume around half of their diet as carbohydrates. This comes from rice, wheat, bread, potatoes, pasta, macaroni etc.

## Protein

Proteins are the main tissue builders in the body. They are part of every cell in the body. Proteins help in cell structure, functions, and hemoglobin formation to carry oxygen, enzymes to carry out vital reactions and a myriad of other functions in the body. Proteins are also vital in supplying nitrogen for DNA and RNA genetic material and energy production.

Proteins are necessary for nutrition because they contain amino acids. Among the 20 or more amino acids, the human body is unable to synthesize 8 and these are called essential amino acids.

The essential amino acids include lysine, tryptophan, methionine, leucine, isoleucine, phenylalanine, valine, and threonine.

## Fat

Fats are concentrated sources of energy. They produce an amount of energy twice as carbohydrates or proteins on a weight basis.

The functions of fats include:

They help to form the cellular structure; forming a protective cushion and insulation around vital organs; helping absorb fat-soluble vitamins, providing reserve storage for energy. Essential fatty acids include unsaturated fatty acids like linoleic, linolenic, and arachidonic acids. These need to be taken in the diet. Saturated fats, along with cholesterol, have been implicated in arteriosclerosis and heart disease.

## Mineral

The minerals in foods do not contribute directly to energy needs but are important as body regulators and play a role in metabolic pathways of the body. More than 50 elements are found in the human body. About 25 elements have been found to be essential since a deficiency produces specific deficiency symptoms.

Important minerals include calcium, phosphorus, iron, sodium, potassium, chloride ions, copper, cobalt, manganese, zinc, magnesium, fluorine, and iodine."

Source: https://www.news-medical.net/life-sciences/What-is-Metabolism.aspx

**Vitamins** are essential organic compounds that the human body cannot synthesize by itself and must, therefore, be present in the diet. Vitamins particularly important in metabolism include Vitamin A, B2 (riboflavin), Niacin or nicotinic acid, Pantothenic Acid, etc. The chemical reactions of metabolism are organized into metabolic pathways. These allow the basic chemicals from nutrition to be transformed through a series of steps into another chemical, by a sequence of enzymes.

**Enzyme** are crucial to metabolism because they allow organisms to drive desirable reactions that require energy.

# The free radicals

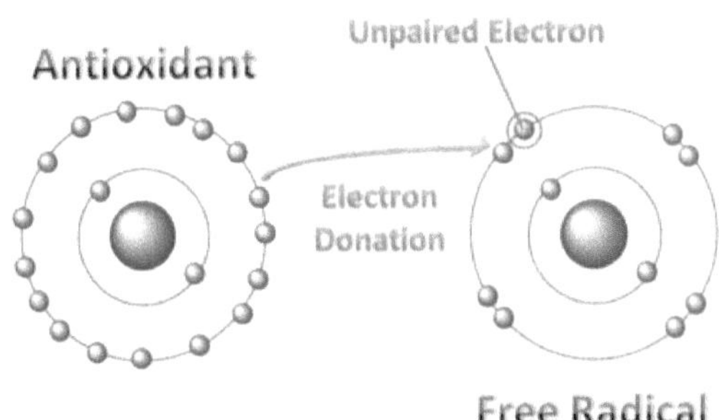



https://en.wikipedia.org/wiki/Amino_radical

To this day, research by scientists has shown that the main culprit of aging and disease is free radicals.

In the chemical structure, electrons tend to bond together so that the outermost electron ring of the atom has eight electrons. Due to chemical or radiation effects, a chemical bond that has two electrons, in the molecule of a substance, is broken, creating two pieces of the molecule. Each piece of the molecule holding an electron to become a free radical. Single, unpaired electrons tend to pair with another electron. Therefore, free radicals have very strong oxidation properties. They always try to get the electrons they lack from other molecules, and consequently, lead to the formation of a series of free radicals.

They react even towards themselves: their molecules will often spontaneously dimerize or polymerize if they come in contact with each other. In chemical equations, free radicals are frequently denoted by a dot placed immediately to the right of the atomic symbol or molecular formula.

Example of a free radical is:

The hydroxyl radical (HO·) is a molecule that has one unpaired electron on the oxygen atom. The two most important oxygen-centered free radicals are superoxides and hydroxyl radicals. They derive from molecular oxygen under reducing conditions.

Chlorine gas can be broken down by ultraviolet light to form atomic chlorine radicals.

Free radicals may be created in a number of ways, including reactions at very low temperatures, or any process that puts enough energy into the parent molecule, such as ionizing radiation, heat, electrical discharges, electrolysis, and chemical reactions, also can affect breakup of larger molecules. Radicals are intermediate stages in many chemical reactions.

The formation of radicals may involve the breaking of covalent bonds by hemolysis, a process that requires significant amounts of energy. Such energies are known as homolytic bond dissociation energies.

The energy needed to break a specific bond (generally covalent) between two atoms known as bond energy. Likewise, radicals requiring more energy to form are less stable than those requiring less energy.

Radical formation through homolytic bond cleavage most often happens between two atoms of similar electronegativity; in organic chemistry, this is often between the O–O bonds in peroxide species or between O–N bonds. Radicals may also be formed by single-electron oxidation or reduction of an atom or molecule.

Free radicals play an important role in many other chemical processes. In living organisms, the free radicals superoxide and nitric oxide and their reaction products regulate many processes, such as control of vascular tone and thus blood pressure. They also play a key role in the intermediary metabolism of various biological compounds.

**In biology**

Because of their reactivity, excessive amounts of these free radicals can lead to cell injury.

In the body, they attack the cell membrane, protein molecules, etc., and the cell nucleus. They cause aging and may also contribute too many diseases such as cancer, stroke, myocardial infarction, diabetes and major disorders. Many forms of cancer are thought to be the result of reactions between free radicals and DNA, potentially resulting in mutations that can adversely affect the cell cycle and potentially lead to malignancy. Some of the symptoms of aging such as atherosclerosis are also attributed to free-radical induced oxidation of cholesterol to 7-ketocholesterol. In addition, free radicals contribute to alcohol-induced liver damage, perhaps more than alcohol itself. Free radicals produced by cigarette smoke are implicated in the inactivation of alpha 1-antitrypsin in the lung. This process promotes the development of emphysema.

"Free radicals may also be involved in Parkinson's disease, senile and drug-induced deafness, schizophrenia, and Alzheimer's.

The classic free-radical syndrome, the iron-storage disease hemochromatosis, often associated with free radical-related symptoms including movement disorder, psychosis, skin pigmentary melanin abnormalities, deafness, arthritis, and diabetes mellitus. The free-radical theory of aging proposes that free radicals underlie the aging process itself."

Source: https://www.news-medical.net/life-sciences/What-is-Metabolism.aspx

Reactive oxygen species (ROS) are species such as superoxide, hydrogen peroxide, and hydroxyl radical, commonly associated with cell damage. ROS is formed as a natural by-product of the normal metabolism of oxygen and has important roles in cell signaling. Oxybenzone has been found to form free radicals in sunlight and therefore may be associated with cell damage. This only occurred when it was combined with other ingredients commonly found in sunscreens, like titanium oxide and octyl methoxycinnamate.

ROS attack the polyunsaturated fatty acid, linoleic acid, to form a series of 13-Hydroxyoctadecadienoic acid and 9-Hydroxyoctadecadienoic acid products that serve as signaling molecules that may trigger responses that counter the tissue injury, which caused their formation. ROS attacks other polyunsaturated fatty acids, e.g. arachidonic acid and docosahexaenoic acid.

***

The body has a number of mechanisms to minimize free-radical-induced damage and to repair the damage that occurs, such as the enzymes superoxide dismutase, catalase, glutathione peroxidase, and glutathione reeducates.

In addition, antioxidants play a key role in these defense mechanisms. These are often the three vitamins, vitamin A, vitamin C, and vitamin E and polyphenol antioxidants. Furthermore, there is good evidence indicating that bilirubin and uric acid can act as antioxidants to help neutralize certain free radicals.

# The protein synthesis in cell

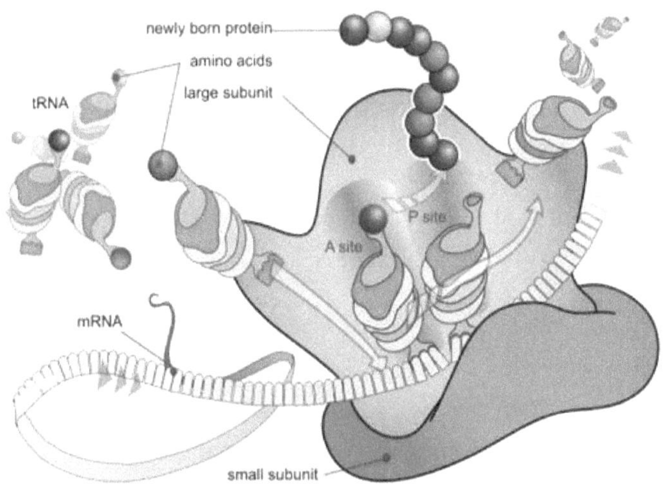



Source:
https://en.wikipedia.org/wiki/Protein_biosynthesis#/media/File:Ribosom e_mRNA_translation_en.svg

Protein biosynthesis is the process whereby biological cells generate new proteins; it is balanced by the loss of cellular proteins. Translation, the assembly of amino acids by ribosomes, is an essential part of the biosynthetic pathway, along with the generation of messenger RNA (mRNA), aminoacylation of transfer RNA (tRNA), co-translational transport, and post-translational modification. Protein biosynthesis is strictly regulated at multiple steps. They are principal during transcription (phenomena of RNA synthesis from DNA template).

Source: https://en.wikipedia.org/wiki/Protein_biosynthesis.

- Translation (phenomena of the amino acid assembly from RNA):

The cistron DNA is transcribed into RNA used as a template in the synthesis of a polypeptide chain.

Protein will often be synthesized directly from genes by translating mRNA.

In protein synthesis, a succession of tRNA molecules charged with appropriate amino acids is brought together with an mRNA molecule and matched up by base-pairing through the anti-codons of the tRNA with successive codons of the mRNA.

The amino acids are then linked together to extend the growing protein chain, and the tRNAs, no longer carrying amino acids, are released.

This whole complex of processes is carried out by the ribosome, formed of two main chains of RNA, called ribosomal RNA (rRNA), and more than 50 different proteins. The ribosome latches onto the end of an mRNA molecule and moves along it, capturing loaded tRNA molecules and joining together their amino acids to form a new protein chain.

(Source: https://en.wikipedia.org/wiki/Protein_biosynthesis)

In the United States, eating habits often use fast food such as chips, hamburgers, poultry, etc. and carbonated beverages. Americans consume too much added sugar, saturated fat, and oil; in contrast, they consume low fruits and vegetables and eat most refined grains. As a result, there are many obese people in the US and many people with cardiovascular disease and cancer.

According to Centers Disease Control and Prevention:

*"Heart disease is the leading cause of death for men, women, and people of most racial and ethnic groups in the United States.*

*One person dies every 37 seconds in the United States from cardiovascular disease.*

*About 647,000 Americans die from heart disease each year—that's in every 4 deaths.*

*Heart disease costs the United States about $219 billion each year from 2014 to 2015. This includes the cost of health care services, medicines, and lost productivity due to death."*

(Source: https://www.cdc.gov/heartdisease/facts.htm)

According to the American Cancer Society:

*"In 2019, there will be an estimated 1,762,450 new cancer cases diagnosed and 606,880 cancer deaths in the United States."*

(Source: https://www.cancer.org/research/cancer-facts-statistics/all-cancer-facts-figures/cancer-facts-figures-2019.html)

American Institute for Cancer Research (AICR) advised people to be vegetarian to prevent cancer, mainly to eat seeds, nuts, beans, grain products, fruits, vegetables, and some animal foods. This will provide the body with anti-cancer active ingredients such as phytochemicals, vitamins, minerals, and fiber.

*"AICR recommends that you fill your plate with 2/3 (or more) plant foods and 1/3 (or less) fish, poultry or meat, and dairy."*

https://www.aicr.org/patients-survivors/healthy-or-harmful/vegetarian-and-vegan.html

According to a Harris Interactive poll conducted by the Vegetarian Resource Group, approximately six to eight million adults in the United States eat no meat, fish, or poultry.

Traditionally, researchers have suggested that the vegetarian diet is nutritionally deficient, but in recent years, they are confirming that eating without meat will have health benefits. Vegetarians are not only provided with adequate nutrients but also prevent many chronic diseases.

*"Compared with meat eaters, vegetarians tend to consume less saturated fat and cholesterol and more vitamins C and E, dietary fiber, folic acid, potassium, magnesium, and phytochemicals (plant chemicals), such as carotenoids and flavonoids. As a result, they're likely to have lower total and LDL (bad) cholesterol, lower blood pressure, and lower body mass index (BMI), all of which are associated with longevity and a reduced risk for many chronic diseases."*

https://www.health.harvard.edu/staying-healthy/becoming-a-vegetarian

# DISCUSSION

The human body synthesizes many amino acids, only does not synthesize the essential amino acids. Therefore, these acids need to be provided from the food source. The body's cells use amino acids from the food source to synthesize proteins for various body functions. Depending on the different functions of the cell types, they have different lifetimes.

There are long living cells: Lymphocytes: from 2 months to 1 year; Red blood cells: 4 months; Macrophages: from 1 month to 1 year; Endothelial cells: from 1 month to 1 year; Pancreas: 1 year or more; Bones: 25 to 30 years. In a mature man, the liver replaces itself about once a year to five and a half. The entire human skeleton is supposed to be replaced every 10 years or so in adults.

Therefore, people eat meat every day, often resulting in excess protein compared to the body's needs. This excess is main the source of nutrition for the cancerous tumors of the sick. If cancer patients eat proteins from plants sources instead of animal proteins, this harmful excess would be avoided because proteins from plants usual contain a low percentage of the essential amino acids.

If the supply lacks any essential amino acids, cancer cells will not be able to synthesize proteins to develop tumors. It will die!

That is the most important scientific nature of using vegetarianism to cure cancer that the author wants to explain and prove in this book.

DONG LA

# Appendix

## The story about a "Holy Lady" which has a strange ability to cure cancer

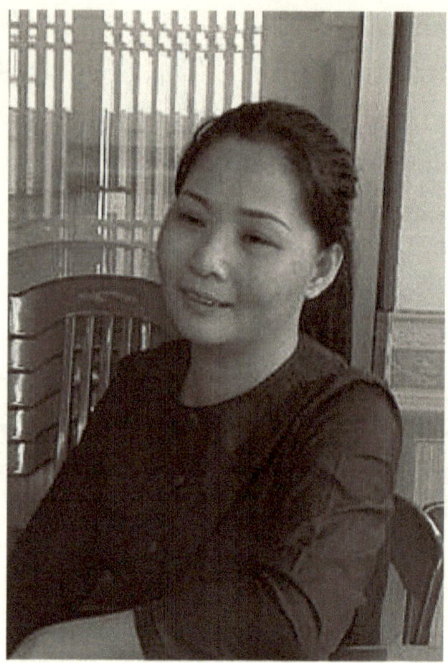

(Mrs. Vu Thi Hoa)

Mrs. Vu Thi Hoa is a woman who has strange abilities. Many people and I have witnessed her strange abilities such as communicating with the souls of the dead, looking through space and time, looking deep underground, and she also helped some people get rid of cancer. For example, she in Hanoi could see me doing something in Saigon and once from Vietnam, she even saw my son very far away in America.

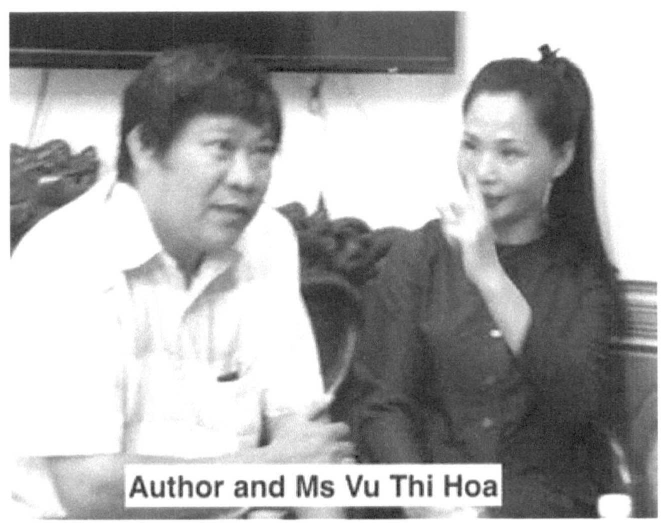

Author and Ms Vu Thi Hoa

I took a lot of pictures of people who were helped spiritually and cured of incurable diseases by her. They kneel down in front of her to give thanks, honoring her as a Bodhisattva:

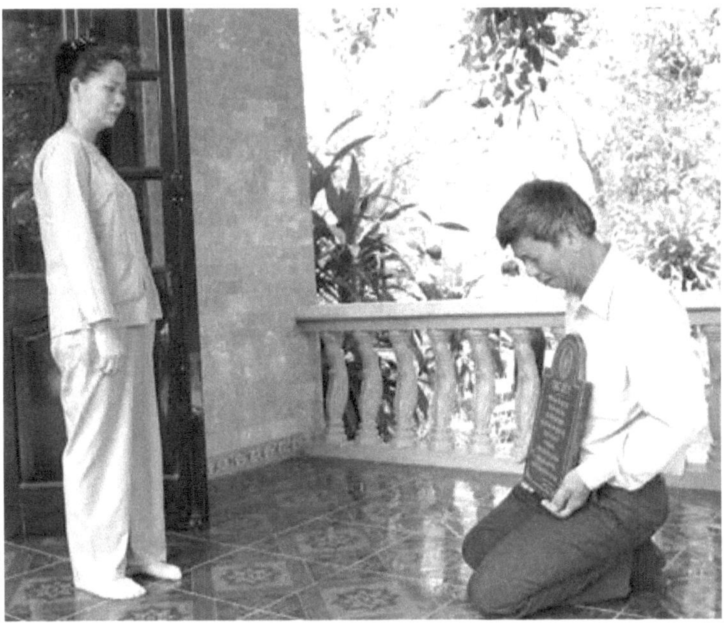

In order to cure the disease, she often gives the patient a drink of coconut water, bottled water, after she has "transmitted energy". She only holds the bottle in her hand; the bottle of water from the normal temperature can be hot to 80-900C. The recipient of the water often said she "bless" them like received "holy water".

She also often uses the medicinal plants in the forest, most notably a root that is not present in any traditional medicine book.

Regarding the ability of Ms. Vu Thi Hoa to treat cancer, I just mention two examples.

1-First is Mrs. Chu Thi Xoan who suffered from brain tumors.

This is the content of the letter that Mrs. Xoan sent to Ms. Vu Thi Hoa:

"Dear Mrs. Vu Thi Hoa!

My name is Chu Thi Xoan,

Address: Hamlet 14, Dang Xa village, Kim Bang district, Ha Nam province.

I write this letter to express the gratitude of a person returning from the dead. Thank you very much for saving me from brain cancer:

The evil illness tortured me. I went to the hospitals to be treated by the doctors, but the doctors were helpless to let me go home waiting die. It was February 15, 2012. After, the pains tormented me, as if my brain was broken. I kept ramming my head against the wall, want the pain outside to reduce the pain inside.

On February 16, 2012, I met you. You looked at me with a compassionate look. You have the compassion of Avalokitesvara Bodhisattva rescuing the human. You accept healing for me. You give me three fruits of coconuts; I drink every time one fruit. Drinking the first fruit, I feel the pain decreased. Drinking the second fruit, the pain more decreased. Drinking the third fruit, like a miracle, the pain gradually disappeared.

Luckily, I met you. Now, I do not know what to do to repay you; I only thank you very much!

On January 15, 2013, I met the doctor; He concluded that I was cured. Now, I return to normal life and go back to work as before.

Chu Thi Xoan

2- Mrs. Truong Thi Ngoc Minh:

This woman lives in Vung Tau. In 2009, when she came to the hospital, the doctors diagnosed her with stage 2-bladder cancer.

After that, she had surgery twice and was given chemotherapy to prevent metastases. In August 2011, Mrs. Minh met Mrs. Vu Thi Hoa. Mrs. Hoa looked at Mrs. Minh's weak body and said, "I will cure you of this illness with my medication. It is important that you have to believe and have to take your medication regularly."

Mrs. Minh was very happy. She did exactly what Mrs. Hoa told her and had a very unexpected result. She felt her health gradually improved. After 4 months of using plant medicine, which Mrs. Hoa gave for her, Mrs. Minh came to the Binh Dan Hospital in Ho Chi Minh City; the doctor said she was cured.

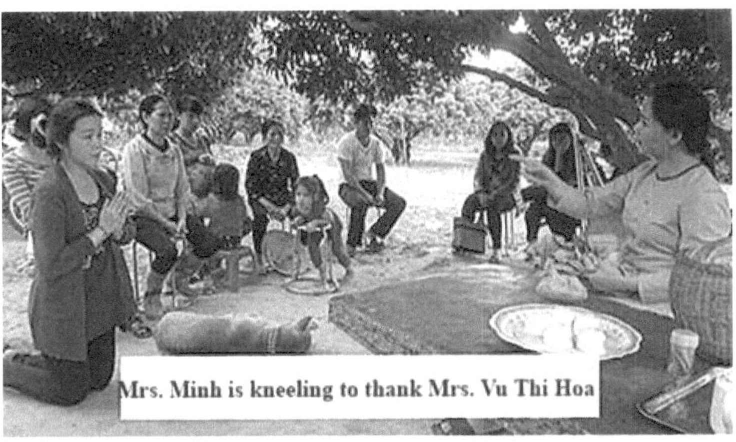


To September 2015, Mrs. Minh once again worried about the recurrence of bladder cancer. After the examination at Binh Dan hospital, the doctor said, she must be operated and radiotherapy because the disease has spread.

At that time, Mrs. Hoa was in Ho Chi Minh City. With the ability to see from afar, Mrs. Hoa knew that Mrs. Minh had recurrent cancer. She phoned Mrs. Minh, told Mrs. Minh coming to meet her right away.

Then, within 4 months, Mrs. Minh came to Vinh Phuc, where Mrs. Hoa lived, to cure. In early 2016, she returned home in a happy mood. Because on August 12, 2016, she went to see a doctor, again the doctors, after the examination, said she was cured!

However, not everyone with cancer can be cured by Mrs. Hoa. This is also a mystery in the spiritual world.

***

The stories about Mrs. Vu Thi Hoa are like legends, but all are the true. I was once a researcher in pharmaceutical chemistry and also a writer, critic, so I'm not superstitious. Writing about her, I just want to say that life has a lot of mystery beyond the vision of science. As in modern medicine, many people still do not believe in vegetarian diets that can cure cancer, but it is true.

Ho Chi Minh City, Vietnam

February 1, 2020


ĐÔNG LA